Arvin Dibra

Network of excellence in surgical research

Arvin Dibra

Network of excellence in surgical research

The SMIT MAP experience

LAP LAMBERT Academic Publishing

Imprint

Any brand names and product names mentioned in this book are subject to trademark, brand or patent protection and are trademarks or registered trademarks of their respective holders. The use of brand names, product names, common names, trade names, product descriptions etc. even without a particular marking in this work is in no way to be construed to mean that such names may be regarded as unrestricted in respect of trademark and brand protection legislation and could thus be used by anyone.

Cover image: www.ingimage.com

Publisher:
LAP LAMBERT Academic Publishing
is a trademark of
Dodo Books Indian Ocean Ltd. and OmniScriptum S.R.L publishing group

120 High Road, East Finchley, London, N2 9ED, United Kingdom
Str. Armeneasca 28/1, office 1, Chisinau MD-2012, Republic of Moldova, Europe
Managing Directors: Ieva Konstantinova, Victoria Ursu
info@omniscriptum.com

Printed at: see last page
ISBN: 978-3-659-52769-2

Zugl. / Approved by: Rome, Tor Vergata University, 2010

Network of excellence in surgical research.

The SMIT MAP experience.

The writing of a dissertation can be a lonely and isolating experience, yet it is obviously not possible without the personal and practical support of numerous people. Thus my sincere gratitude goes to my dear wife Frida, to my parents and my friends for their love, support, and patience.

Table of contents

Preface

When the scientific collaboration with Prof. Arvin Dibra started, years ago, I have not thought about today, when with great pleasure, I agreed to write a few words as a preface to the publication of his scientific research.

I closely followed up the development of the project, which Mr Dibra has carefully extended in this book, and it is actually very dear to me. What the author argues in this book is instinctively what, all together with my SMIT colleagues, we imagined when deciding to kick off the project of SMIT MAP.

We created a peculiar network, that can accommodate anyone who has the same objective, meaning producing technological innovation of excellence applied to medicine, and more precisely to the surgical sciences.

I am really happy to present this book, where the reader will learn not only how our platform of excellence was born, but will also have useful information on the process of setting innovation technology applied to surgery, and on the needs that give rise to and evolve constantly.

Not as a second endpoint, the book also describes the most recent thinking wave on how technology can find the best conditions to give the best contributions to medical progress, by refining what already exists or by creating useful innovations that until recently remained in the clouds of science fiction .

Finally, I think that this book and its author deserve the best consideration from the scientific community for this excellent scientific contribute.

Nicola Di Lorenzo, MD, PhD, FACS

Associate Professor of General Surgery

Past President (2005) of SMIT (Society for Medical Innovations and Technology)

Past Chairman (2009-13) Of The Technology Committee OF EAES (European Association For Endoscopic Surgery)

President 2014-16 of SICOB (Società Italiana di Chirurgia dell'Obesità e delle Malattie Metaboliche)

Director of PhD on Innovative technologies and Medical Engineering for Surgery

Dept. Of Experimental Medicine and Surgery - Università di Roma Tor Vergata

Prelude

Perhaps to all of you who hand a writing of some years ago, the memory of those old pages fades away and is locked in some precious moment of your life. What happened to me was not only a revival of old times, but also a source of pride when the publisher of the book that you have in your hands today, came with a proposal to publish what had been my doctoral research. It happened that I felt totally undecided whether should I change the opinions expressed and update them with actuals facts, or should I hand over the work as it was, leaving the dignity and simplicity to the reflections, experiences and collaborations that I had at that time. And, perhaps, the collaborations were an essential part when trying to find the thread of need, or better to say, the necessity to have a network when you try to make innovation in surgery. In *fact*, I was doing my own *thinking* all the time, long before I started to write something down a paper or a book in which everything could be expressed, thrown out of my mind, changed, modified or remained still the same over the argument. Just as often this thought was removed, flushed by a multitude of jobs commitments that the urgency of their pitch took out all the spare time.

During these years, I often had the opportunity to observe the extraordinary importance of collaboration between people in surgery and instinctively, I was thinking about the very necessity of networking among specialized centers in order to produce new instruments or to optimize existing ones in this ordeal profession. At the same thoughts my instinct has led flounder during long and strenuous efforts to make some scientific research with the few tools that may have a professional living and working for several years in an emerging country with poor economy. After so long, I concluded that it is just the cooperation network that may have the right chance and satisfaction of proving any achievement, no matter how small, into a specific chain of research. Cooperation networks should consist of different research centers and would be comprising researchers like me and my colleagues with a strong inventive and rich in desire but rather poor in resources. In this way, the theory of the network of excellence and the possibility of involvement for scientists that work in emerging countries, became one of the focal points of my lectures that I had the opportunity to give as guest professor at the Doctoral School of the University of Rome "Tor Vergata", during the doctoral lectures on the use of advanced technology in emerging countries.

It happens to any researcher to be divided between the daily commitments that are constantly filled with deadlines and the feeling that many of your reflections still need more experience to be crystallized clearly in a book another, so I decided to confine myself to these few introductory words, leaving to the future the opportunity to do something more. In conclusion, a special thank you is reserved for the Publisher. I would like to thank you for the smooth publication of this writings and to have found enough value in them to give the light of print. On these pages are impressed many pleasant memories filled with the pure enthusiasm of a young man who begins his journey in science among adults. This trip has been a kind endevour with all those friends for which is written in this book. Hence, in these lines I want to conclude by expressing my thanks to all the staff of SMIT MAP creators for the great opportunity they gave me, to all those who gave me the opportunity to meet and observe closely the way that were built serious consortium as VEKTOR and ARAKNES and where, to my very pleasant surprise, one of the originators and main actors of these projects, Prof. Marc Schurr, a global example of knowledge that constantly produces surgical technological innovation, was also part of the final evaluation commission of my dissertation. I wish to thank Prof. Achille Lucio Gaspari and my esteemed advisor and supervisor, Prof. Nicola Di Lorenzo, for inspiring and encouraging me to pursue a career in Research in Surgical Innovations and for enabling me to do so.

My research would not have been possible without the expert guidance of Prof. Alberto Arezzo the ideator and founder of the SMIT MAP. Not only was he readily available for me, but he always read and responded to my questions more quickly than I could have hoped. And above all the qualities and flaws that certainly bears these writings, this evaluation was certainly an additional motive of satisfaction, which I wuold like to share with all of you who started the long and difficult road of surgery.

Introduction

Incremental innovation in biomedical devices is relatively straightforward. Today's product line gets upgraded to become smaller, faster, cheaper, etc – but there's little fundamental change to underlying technologies, clinical procedures, health service provision, regulatory requirements, and so on. Unfortunately incremental innovations are insufficient in today's fast-moving world, and all interested in recognising the need to invest in more disruptive innovation if they are to protect and grow their research and businesses.

It is hard for a single centre or company to identify and capture the disruptive opportunities that arise at the interfaces between clinical procedures and research into medicine, biology, engineering and physics and mostly it is even often very risky. The purpose of the excellence platform we are presenting is to create a dedicated process, organisation and network that binds together researchers from across these disciplines with clinicians, health service providers, biomedical device companies and funders/investors, to identify and rapidly implement mutually beneficial opportunities.

Clinical needs are the key drivers for Smit Map Network of Excellence. The Society for Medical Innovations and Technology (SMIT) is an international society, formed in 1989 under the name "Society for Minimally Invasive Therapy" by an innovative group of medical practitioners led by John Wickham. The founding members were leaders in their fields and were dedicated to the multidisciplinary advancement of minimally invasive therapy in an attempt to reduce patient trauma arising from surgical operations or radiological interventions. The current membership base includes representatives from most medical specialities, instrument manufacturing, biomedical engineering and research. As to reflect this broader membership as well to attract further members not necessarily only within minimally invasive therapy, the name of the Society was formally changed to "Society for Medical Innovation and Technology" during the 12th Congress in the year 2000.

In the year 2006 the Steering Committee of the Society decided to create a Network of Excellence, named SMIT MAP. Its role is to assemble the right collaborations and knowledge exchange around the right opportunities and ensure a smooth path from lab to clinic.

The areas where recent scientific discoveries promise valuable advances for patients, healthcare providers and life science companies alike are: Diagnostic & therapeutic imaging; Drug delivery: Regenerative medicine; Robotics in surgical techniques; Minimally Invasive therapy tools and Tissue Ablation Interface translational science – the convergence of traditional scientific disciplines – is the key to today's major medical advances and innovations. Experts within the medical, physical and biological sciences experts from the departments of many well-known Universities in the world have been working like this for years – pooling their talents and resources on world-class research of enormous benefit to 21st century healthcare.

The aim is to put engineers, physicists, mathematicians and life scientists together with clinicians, health service providers, and corporates to research and exploit the developments that are occurring at the interface between the biomedical and physical sciences. Our Network is a single, dedicated organisation with the vision, collaborative ethos and resources to make it happen.

An effective research and standardized development process is absolutely central to SMIT MAP's success and will be necessary continue to invest heavily in this aspect.

Smit Map will be a tool of cooperation between research centres, health service providers and corporate partners at all stages, from early stage scientific research to the development of specific biomedical devices. The Network can become the tool to complete the transfer of development activities to the corporate partner(s) activities during the Pre-Clinical Trials Phase of the process.

Certification of partners development processes (ISO, GLP, etc.) will facilitate the efficient, economic transfer of new device technologies to the corporate partners.

The partners in this Network can conduct world-class research and development in several areas promising valuable advances for patients, healthcare providers and life science companies alike.

Independently, the actual SMIT partners have enviable reputations in the fields of medicine, physics and the biological sciences.

Much of these partners are acknowledged centre of excellence in physics research and a focal point for medical research. Others, with its eminent Schools of Medicine, Life Sciences and Engineering, and Ninewells Teaching Hospital (part of the European and North American realities), a community of knowledge has grown up in the last years that offers unique scientific and commercial opportunities to make far-reaching advances in diagnosis and treatment. Add all them together represent a formidable bank of research excellence, clinical expertise and application development - a force with the potential to create world-class research of enormous benefit to 21st century healthcare.

The outcomes will:

· Enhanced basic/applied research agendas, with long-term efforts directed to real clinical and patient needs

· Ideas for new biomedical device concepts to put into our development pipeline

Biomedical device concepts can be taken through the different centres structured development process by a cross-functional team of scientists, engineers, clinicians, and business developers. Team members can drawn from the partners to ensure coordinated assessment and development of clinical, commercial and technical aspects. At some point in the development process, leadership is transferred to a corporate partner – be this a spin-out business, or an existing medical device / life science company – to complete the journey to the market place.

Chapter 1

How SMIT MAP was born…

Sometime between antiquity and the late 19th and early 20th century, the favored form of surgical intervention transformed into one dominated by big incisions. Exploratory laparotomies eventually came to be understood as integral to the treatment and diagnosis of many types of disease states that had defied other methods of diagnosis. Ironically, this growing preference for "classical" open surgery was most likely influenced significantly by the scientific advances in asepsis and anesthesia during the same time period, discoveries which finally ushered in the era of modern medicine.

With the advent of anesthesia and antiseptic however, this meant that for the first time in living patients the physician could now get right to the source of disease without having to rely on deductive reasoning or blind biopsies. Diseases of the abdomen could now be palpated, visualized, and treated surgically. Paradoxically then, while treatment options and recovery rates expanded, so too did the circumference of incisions. Open approaches were soon codified as the gold standards of "classical surgery," a point that later served to interfere substantially with endoscopy's progress .

Taken collectively, these great strides in medicine, coupled with parallel advances in science and technology so characteristic of this late Industrial era, engendered a growing sense of scientific infallibility.

Traditional surgical conventions continued to undergo rapid change as well. Many snappy aphorisms from our not too distant past supported this growing reverence for surgeons and by extension, for their surgical procedures too. Such sayings as "to cut is to cure," "the greater the surgeon, bigger the incision".

Influenced by this entrenched dogma, the inherent morbidity associated with large incisions was de-emphasized, due mainly to the lack of surgical alternatives. Contrary to today's standards, a large incision was seen as a necessary evil, unequivocally required to save the life of the patient.

Of course, the sacrosanct system of scientific lore is often paradoxically unwelcoming of new-fangled notions, subjecting novel ideas to sometimes rancorous resistance. Our discipline clearly witnessed such a backlash to new ideas when we saw, for instance, operative videolaparoscopy so vehemently lambasted in its early ascendancy. Indeed, videolaparoscopy, by catalyzing such profound changes to the very foundation of so-called "classical" surgery, came to symbolize an unwelcome threat to the entire order of things.

The lowest birth rates and fastest growing elderly population in the advanced industrial world, there is great concern over raising health costs in the years ahead. To deal with this emerging situation, every effort must be made to prevent disease in the first place, but when medical conditions do arise, it is of course desirable that patients recover and return to work as quickly as possible. This makes it all the more urgent to establish medical procedures that minimize pain and trauma to patients, and to develop advanced clinical systems that support those ends. The medical equipment industry has seen rapid development of sophisticated diagnostic systems that exploit the rapid advances of information technology. Therapeutic systems have also benefited and shown enormous progress over the last few years by leveraging the advances in imaging and robotics technologies.

The advent of minimally invasive surgery and the resulting boundaries for the surgeon due to the length of the instruments, reduction in degrees of freedom, 2D image, and lack of haptics, called on robots to improve these limitations and they once again appeared to show potential. Today, with the broader availability of robots, more and more surgeons are evaluating their clinical significance in a wide range of surgeries. Furthermore, uncharted areas of image-guided surgery, preplanning and automation are once again of interest to researchers and to industry. Telepresence surgery also continues to garner significant interest and there are ongoing investments for research in this field. In the distant future, there will be semi-autonomous and autonomous systems which the surgeon will program and will be executed precisely by intelligent computer-assisted/robotic systems. But more important, clinical practice and research will move more to interdisciplinary approach, using biology, physics (engineering) and informatics to create devices and methods that are even less invasive, more precise, and more cost effective. The power of biology (flexible, adaptable, self-assembling and self-maintaining) with engineering (robust, accurate, powerful) and informatics (intelligent, networked, wireless) will result in intelligent systems which act non-invasively at the point of care. The surgeon will still have procedures that are hands-on, especially the more complex procedures, and will be replacing organs with synthetic, artificial organs off the shelf - a combination of manufactured and biologically grown. Surgical instruments will be "smart", using micro-electro-mechanical systems (MEMS) and nanotechnology to provide haptics and other information directly to the surgeon's hand.

With these assumptions was founded in 1989 the Society for Medical Innovations and Technology is an international society under the name "Society for Minimally Invasive Therapy" SMIT by an innovative group of medical practitioners led by John Wickham. The founding members were leaders in their fields and were dedicated to the multidisciplinary advancement of minimally invasive therapy in an attempt to reduce patient trauma arising from surgical operations or radiological interventions. The current membership base includes representatives from most medical specialities, instrument manufacturing, biomedical engineering and research.

As to reflect this broader membership as well to attract further members not necessarily only within minimally invasive therapy, the name of the Society was formally changed to "Society for Medical Innovation and Technology" during the 12th Congress in the year 2000.

Linking institutions based in different countries and even on different continents resulted in the development of several common concepts, methods, instruments and standards as well as common publications – an output much more extensive than what might have been accomplished in research done by each single institution on its own.

SMIT over the years has seen the addition of new members bringing together in the same society so many important research centres experts in design, realization and clinical application of innovative new methods and advanced technologies.

SMIT principal activity is reflected annually now for 21 years in international conferences where are published and discussed the important progress made by individual centres or by cooperation between several members.

Between them we can find some academic centres focused in development of interdisciplinary research combining Physical Sciences and Engineering with Biology and Medicine integrating basic science together with clinical and industrial applications. Their objectives include molecular and cellular structure and functions research using micro and nano-technologies, and the development of microsystems to integrate detection and micromanipulation at the molecular and cellular scale.

The research objectives are the development and application of technologies at the micro and scale to obtain basic knowledge and technological applications in the emergent areas of Biophysics and Bioengineering. Moreover, it is also essential to educate new scientists in this interdisciplinary area. As a consequence of the research tasks, those centers promotes knowledge and technology transfer to other groups in biomedical research and to close industrial sectors as the pharmaceutical and medical technologies.

A further objective is that one to participate also in SMIT professional research companies for the healthcare operating on an international basis and maintaining a well-established network of partners in leading scientific institutions. They support manufacturers and users of medical products and services in all aspects , such as research, design, product assessment and marketing.

In their projects they use well-defined, highly developed methods, from the analysis of market requirements and competition, to product definition, up to experimental research in laboratories. Some of them invest also in start-up companies and help to convert their technological competence into business success.

This clear profile and long term experience in the management of innovation make those companies professional partners of business and science on an international scale.

SMIT also participate many centers for production of medical instruments and materials that with their important research centers and their high production capacity become important partners of the area of scientific interest and application.

Over the years of the association many of these participants have a long and interesting history of cooperation between them. These collaborations are in the years to become stable and have given good results in many cases of scientific work. There have been some great assessments on these collaborations of international scientific opinion and a large interest of the industry of medical devices. We can mention here some joint projects that have had the approval and funding from the European Commission and which still continue their scientific research with good results. They are the VECTOR Project (IST-2005-2.5.2; EU 033970) and the ARAKNES Project (ICT- 2007.3.6; EU 224565).

In this context a group of SMIT partners has designed and begun work to build a network of excellence called SMIT Map.

SMIT Map today is an updated list of selected research center in the field of new technologies applied to medicine. It is open to Institutions, Schools, Companies, Foundations, and which ever entity produces research in the field of new technologies applied to medicine.

The ambitious aim of this project is to function as an ideal bridge between health care providers at the front line of patient care and operators engaged in the revolution in medical innovations, research and production in Diagnostic & therapeutic imaging; Drug delivery: Regenerative medicine; Robotics in surgical techniques; Minimally Invasive therapy tools and Tissue Ablation. The network tries to centralize new knowledge in one forum to give a quick and comprehensive explication over new innovations and relevant research.

The scope is to advance the quickly developing field of new techniques and innovations in a more and more technically demanding field. It offers an opportunity.

We recognize the need for a dynamic forum that fosters the exchange of ideas across the entire community working in these areas.

Chapter 2

Why do we need a Excellence Network…

In the final years of the XXth century we entered a knowledge-based society. Economic and social development will depend essentially on knowledge in its different forms, on the production, acquisition and use of knowledge. Scientific research and technological development more particularly are at the heart of what makes society tick.

More and more, activities undertaken in this domain are for the express purpose of meeting a social demand and satisfying social needs, especially in connection with the evolution of work and the emergence of new ways of life and activities.

By creating new products, processes and markets research and technology provide one of the principal driving forces of economic growth, competitiveness and employment. They are the best way of modernising companies, which must do to improve its competitive position. In overall terms, both directly and indirectly, they help to maintain and develop employment.

By way of example: The European Council has stressed on several occasions in recent years the importance of sustained research and technological development for growth and employment. The European Parliament, for its part, has often drawn attention to the need for Europe to increase investment in science and technology.

Mapping of European centres of excellence would make for better transparency in this area. A very high level of performance could also be achieved by the networking of specialist centres throughout the countries of the Union. The forms of teleworking which electronic networks permit make it possible to create real "virtual centres of excellence", in particular multidisciplinary and involving universities and companies.

To promote excellence, however, it is also necessary to ensure a sufficient level of competition between private and public research operators. Schemes to finance centres of excellence on the basis of competition have been put in place in several Member States. This formula could be applied to the European level, with collaboration between the Commission and the Member States.

A central feature of actor-network theory is that humans and non-humans (technology, organizations, institutions, etc.) are treated symmetrically. Technological and social elements are considered tied together into networks, based on the assumption that technologies are always defined to work in an environment including non-technological elements, without which the technology would be meaningless and it would not work.

In the same way, as humans, we use non-human objects (technologies and other artefacts) in all our dealings in our world; our existence in the world is based upon the existence of these objects. Accordingly, neither humans nor technological artefacts should be considered as pure, isolated elements, but rather as heterogeneous networks.

When any actor acts, this very actor is always such a network, not a single element. An actor is always a hybrid collective. In the same way, elements in a network are not defined only by their "internal" aspects, but rather by their relationships to other elements, as a network. This further implies that elements in such a network are not initially defined as human, social or technological; they are referred to by a common term: actor. These assumptions do not deny any differences or borders between what is human or social and what is technological.

However, these borders are seen as negotiated, not as given.

According to actor network theory, stability, technological and social order, is continually negotiated as a social process of aligning interests. As actors from the outset have a diverse set of interests, stability rests crucially on the ability to translate (reinterpret, represent, or appropriate) others' interests to one's own.

Through translations, one and the same interest or anticipation may be presented in different ways, thereby mobilizing broader support.

A translation presupposes a medium or a "material into which it is inscribed." Translations are "embodied in texts, machines, bodily skills [which] become their support, their more or less faithful executive".

Design is then a process where various interests are translated into technological solutions as well as organizational arrangements and procedures to be followed to make the technology work properly. In this process, existing technology will be reinterpreted and translated into new ways of using it.

To make the technology work, all these elements must be aligned, i.e., cooperating toward a common goal. This is achieved through a translation process, which, if successful, may lead to alignment.

An aligned network is in a kind of equilibrium or stable state (at least temporarily). The alignment attempts occur through enrolling the different and heterogeneous actors in this network by translating their interests. As large actor-networks are aligned, they may become irreversible and hard to change. The natural starting point for an analysis of the introduction and adaptation of the technology and the organization is to focus on the *work that is required* in order to facilitate the meeting between the technology and the work practices.

In actor-network terms, a "successful" implementation is *a stabilized network*, where the actors are aligned.

The medical work practice has its demands to an acceptable or desirable state of affairs, but so has the technology.

These different demands may peacefully coexist in a stable network, or they may initially be in conflict and thus require "translation work" in order to enrol and align the different actors into the same stable and working network. The situatedness and emergent character of the mutual learning process is evident. Most of it is unplanned and it occurs in real life and in practical use situations, that is transmissions. This emergent character of the process, together with its openness and dependence on adjacent networks, also implies lack of control, and studying most examples we can show the fragility and vulnerability of the achieved alignment.

Several countries in recent decades have claimed national network programs for research in medicine and technological innovations aimed at particularity applied to research and production in Diagnostic & therapeutic imaging; Drug delivery: Regenerative medicine; Robotics in surgical techniques; Minimally Invasive therapy tools and Tissue Ablation Between them, over the European Community mentioned above we can see important programs of this kind in Canada, the United States and Asian realities with the fast development in recent times.

As an example we mentioned the Canadian National Program Networks of Excellence

That program would revolutionize the way Canadians conduct research and train students for the challenges of the knowledge economy, and apply discoveries and technologies to advance the prosperity and quality of life in our nation.

Established by the Government of Canada in 1989, the NCE Program was hailed as an innovative model to link research and development with wealth creation.

The program was aimed at mobilizing the best talent in the academic, private, and voluntary sectors, and applying it to the task of developing the economy and improving the quality of life of Canadians.

Today, the Program remains a key component of the Government Innovation Agenda. It is a program that engages researchers, partners, and institutions in nationwide networks, and that works with users in industry and government to create commercial opportunities and develop public policy based on sound evidence. A precursor to several other initiatives, the NCE Program has helped transform the research landscape and turn country into a global scientific powerhouse.

With its focus on excellence, collaboration, and common vision, the NCE Program has provided the opportunity to bridge disciplines, sectors, and institutions. It has also helped to strengthen in ways never seen before the ability to advance and apply knowledge for the economic and social well- being.

The success of this NCE Program is deeply rooted in the culture of excellence that exists at most universities. It is also the result of the sustained investment by the federal granting agencies-the Natural Sciences and Engineering Research Council, the Canadian Institutes of Health Research (formerly the Medical Research Council), and the Social Sciences and Humanities Research Council.

Thanks to the high standards they have nurtured over the years, the granting councils have made it possible to launch an excellence-based program that would mobilize researchers in every province.

In 2004, this NCE Program brought together 21 networks representing more than 7,000 people, 1300 Canadians organizations in academia and the public and private sectors, and almost 350 international collaborating organizations. Working in multidisciplinary teams, researchers and partners are taking up complex challenges and turning discoveries into economic and social benefits in areas of strategic importance.

Many examples exist in medical research today, of successful networks of excellence. Some of these were created in the form of associations of professionals in one or more medical specialties in order to exchange experience and opinions both in research to clinical practice.

We mentioned E.C.T.A., Eurasian Colorectal Technologies Association who's work at promoting and teaching the use, and discouraging abuse of advanced technologies for both, diagnosis and treatment of large bowel diseases. That association work in strict cooperation with existing national and international societies operating in the same field. With the aims to gather in association doctors and surgeons of European and Asian countries, to encourage and promote scientific and cultural exchange between them with most attention of surgical training research and updating technology creating centres of excellence and a Network between them.

They organize International meetings every two years and support the creation and recognition of Specialization Schools in Colorectal Surgery in the participant countries.

One other way to create scientific networks of excellence can be seen in EURON's (European Robotic Research Networks) experience.

Composed by a community of more than 200 people with a common interest: robots. Its purpose is to bring together the best groups and resources in research, industry and education in Europe and to demonstrate Europe's world class position in robotics. Scientists, industrialists and educators work together towards the dream of the next generation of robots. It is about networking, providing a forum for members to meet and exchange news and results. From this existing friendships are strengthened so that new ideas and collaborations are born, and old ideas are reviewed and extended.

EURON helps to focus European research efforts towards more productive goals. This happens partly through its community activities which allow to exchange ideas and techniques, and partly through identifying the topics where research efforts are best spent and advertising them to scientists and policy-makers.

Believing that new skilled researchers, innovators, engineers and teachers are needed, an aim of that network is to develop and train this new skilled workforce through general science promotion activities and advanced summer schools.

Besides they actively encourages the exchange of ideas and people between the research and industrial communities so that each can benefit from the expertise of the other.

But creating Networks is not a prerogative of developed countries. Same kind of organizations but with other aims are present in different realities.

European and Developing Countries Clinical Trials Partnership EDCTP is currently part of the European Commission's Framework Program for research and technological development aims through research integration to accelerate the development of new or improved drugs, vaccines, diagnostics and microbicides against HIV/AIDS, malaria and tuberculosis, with a focus on phase II and III clinical trials in sub-Saharan Africa.

The countries of Central Africa have joined forces to enable the region to build research capacity and conduct clinical trials under best practices. CANTAM (Central Africa Network on Tuberculosis, HIV/AIDS and Malaria for the conduct of clinical trials) is the first EDCTP-funded regional Network of Excellence to prepare the region to conduct high-quality clinical trials. It will be supported by a grant for the duration of three years. The network includes research institutions and political partners from Cameroon, Congo, Gabon, Tanzania and Germany. It is envisaged that the networks for Eastern, Western and Southern Africa will start their activities later this year.

The number of clinical trials on HIV/AIDS, tuberculosis and malaria conducted in Africa is increasing sharply and is expected to further increase in the coming years. The question is whether the countries of sub-Saharan Africa have sufficient clinical trials centers that are well equipped and staffed to ensure that these trials are conducted according to internationally acceptable standards.

EDCTP therefore set up a grant program to fund regional Networks of Excellence, in which clinical trial centers from various African countries in Central, Eastern, Southern and Western Africa are interlinked at regional level, so that they can complement each other in building capacity to design and conduct large multi-centre clinical trials on HIV/AIDS, tuberculosis and malaria and other related diseases. Ultimately, the four networks will also work in collaboration and complement each other.

The CANTAM is the first network that will start on a regional level to develop capacities in the areas of good clinical and laboratory practice, data management, quality control, and ethics among others. The network includes partner institutions from Cameroon, Congo, Gabon, Tanzania and Germany.

At last we believe the NCE has profoundly transformed the way research is done in universities and has pioneered innovative ways to translate research into economic growth and social progress. By bringing together research and collaboration, networks provide an internationally competitive environment for researchers, clinicians and students to work together with industry, and accelerate the exchange of knowledge and new technology to the private sector.

The launch of the NCE Programs by the European Commission's Framework Programs and similar in other countries set in motion a significant cultural shift within world's research community. By breaking down the barriers between people, disciplines, institutions, and sectors, those programs challenge researchers and their partners to embrace collaboration, multidisciplinarity, and linkages to build a critical mass of expertise in research areas of strategic importance. Collaboration among researchers from different disciplines help to enhance the scope of research topics while providing fresh insight into old problems. Collaboration between researchers and partners provide new opportunities to undertake complex research projects, and to determine at the planning stage how the research results could be used for the people benefit. The researchers' recognition of the opportunities that exist by working with industry proved to be one of the earliest benefits of the NCE. Researchers start thinking in new ways about the problems industry would bring to their attention. For others, the NCE provide an opportunity to focus their research in terms of the needs of industry. Increasingly, researchers became aware of how sponsors could benefit from their work and saw the full potential of talking and interacting with partners and potential users of the research. From an industry perspective, the NCE provide the opportunity to gain immediate access to expertise and research, and to decide on research priorities together with the best scientists and engineers. In the NCE model, partners and research users take part in the management of the networks and in the selection of research projects they undertake. By fostering the efficient and timely sharing of ideas, knowledge, and technology, the NCE programs enables partners to directly benefit from their investment in research. It also gives them a better understanding of future directions and the potential impact of cutting-edge research on their area of activity. One of the most visible successes of the networks is the training of highly qualified personnel in areas where skilled and adaptable professionals are often in short supply. Over the years, networks develop strategies and mechanisms to expose graduate students and postdoctoral researchers to multidisciplinary and multi sectorial approaches. The result is that: a pool of highly adaptable people with broad knowledge, multidimensional thinking, and highly developed problem-solving skills. By training people in a world-class research environment, and by encouraging interaction with private and public sector partners, networks are developing the human and intellectual capital needed to bridge the research and its industrial and social applications. In addition to providing trainees with a launch pad to a variety of careers, networks help to retain the highly skilled people who needs to be competitive globally.

Chapter 3
What is the Surgical Innovation?

Over the last decade, the concepts and principles of innovation have largely been defined through research and publication in the business literature. These concepts in innovation may now be applied to other professions.

Surgery, as one of the oldest and most respected fields, built upon continuous innovation, has a unique culture and deep tradition. While some aspects of research in the broad field of innovation are directly applicable to surgery, many unique aspects of our craft and practice require specialized thought. As such, perhaps it is the surgeon's responsibility to describe and study innovation as it applies to our field.

Today our surgeon colleagues will perform thousands operations each day, many in the abdomen, the chest, or the brain. Innovations that took us from then to now can be thought of in several broad categories. While innovation in surgery has a rich tradition, the field and study of surgical innovation are relatively new. An increasing number of surgical leaders think that innovation may be the only way to maintain the quality of their profession. To date, attempts have been made to systematically evaluate broader concepts in technology innovation as they apply to surgery. Within a context of surgical history, specifically that of surgical endoscopy, we have tried to reference current concepts in the broadest context of technology innovation to the field of surgical innovation.

A dialogue on surgical innovation practice and policy builds upon emerging concepts in technology innovation research. A comprehensive evaluation of surgical innovation would include discussion of ethics, economics, policy, and education, all important aspects.

We will focus here on fundamental concepts of how innovation is defined, assessed, critiqued, and encouraged.

Innovation is a broad term defined as the act of introducing something new or the use of a new idea or method. In some instances, it is used synonymously with invention, although innovation is more precisely defined as something thought up or

27

mentally fabricated. Importantly, no technology or its application is entirely new, as no inventor works within a vacuum. All definitions of innovation involve both new ideas and an act of use or practice. The coupling of new ideas and hands-on use is also a central tenet of surgery, partially explaining the historical success of surgeons as innovators and the progress, which their innovation created. These new ideas may come in the form of technology, technique, or a combination. The process by which surgical innovation applies new ideas to "hands on" clinical needs is analogous to the process by which translational research applies basic research to clinical problems.

Research is not the same as innovation. Advancement in the basic sciences, such as immunology, biochemistry, and physiology, represents critically important progress. This research contributes to the fundamental knowledge base and supports future invention. However, basic science research is not the same as innovation as it does not require application or intended use. The distance between the two can be thought of as the translational gap.

Many terms used within innovation research are new or lack universal definitions. Several terms that are representative of concepts important to surgical innovation require definition and clarity. The terms are fundamentally based on technology, market forces, or clinical impact. These terms are not mutually exclusive and often have overlapping meaning.

Technology innovation may be enabling or incremental. Enabling technology refers to an innovation that supports further developments within a field. An enabling procedure similarly supports development of new procedures within a field. For example, instrument sterilization represented an enabling technology as it supported countless advances within surgery. Similarly, vascular anastomotic technique, was an enabling procedure, promoting a series of advances in surgical technique and innovation, from vascular repair to organ transplantation. On the other hand, an incremental technology change is an innovation which marginally improves upon currently available technology and does not lead to a significant technology shift. A new surgical clip with better holding strength and placement characteristics would represent an incremental change.

Over the last decade, a variety of market-based terms have arisen to describe the commercial impact of innovation. A disruptive technology change is defined as an innovation which topples industry leaders, leading to a significant loss in their market share. In surgery, industry leaders may be defined as the large corporations that often determine technology promotion. In a broader interpretation, industry leaders may be clinical leaders within a medical specialty who often determine technology adoption. In this case, specialty market share changes according to patient volume.

Generally, disruptive innovations are technologically straightforward and begin by catering to an emerging market focused on a new set of product attributes. When introduced, the technology is often inferior to the existing options or otherwise undesirable to customers, causing it to be ignored by industry leaders. As the technology develops, the growth curve of the disruptive innovation surpasses its previous competitor within a segment of the market.

As an example, percutaneous transluminal balloon angioplasty in its early development was dangerous and inferior to open coronary artery bypass. However, it ultimately proved to be disruptive within the field of cardiothoracic surgery, causing a shift in market share toward interventional cardiology.

The opposite of a disruptive change is a sustaining technology change. This change is defined as an improvement, generally made by current industry leaders, to maintain the rate of growth within an existing technology niche. The advances may be large and even enabling to new technology or procedures but are not disruptive to existing market forces. An example of a sustaining technology change is the invention of the coronary stent. This was an incremental change that improved outcomes within an existing market but did not topple either corporate or clinical industry leaders.

In evaluating the history of surgical innovation, the existing terms in technology innovation are useful as they define the nomenclature. Indeed, as the field of technology innovation has matured over the last years, many of these terms have only recently been defined and brought into common usage.

It should be recognized that these concepts and terms grew fundamentally out of business analysis to better understand market forces and industry trends. While these concepts represent a foundation, it is clear that physicians and surgeons often have a different view of technology change than corporate executives.

Most surgeons innovate on a daily basis, tailoring therapies and operations to the intrinsic uniqueness of every patient and their disease.

It is the unsolved problem, or the repetitive failures of existing therapies that stimulate surgeons to find a better way.

Throughout history, surgeons have been the most prolific medical device innovators. Our lexicon in innovation must reflect a history that has often been less dependent upon market forces than upon patient outcome, peer review, and peer esteem.

It should be noted that the impetus for surgical innovation may be changing as surgical care and health care, as a whole, are managed with fiscal performance as at least one primary outcome measure.

In examining the history of surgery, surgical nuances are not well described or accounted for in the current innovation literature. The history of surgical innovation has followed an ebb-and-flow pattern. New enabling technology is developed, generally building upon the work of others.

The technology may be slowly or quickly adopted, but ultimately leads to a rapid expansion of medical capabilities and procedures. This rapid expansion leads to a slower period of technology refinement and consolidation of approach. Where initially physicians may try different techniques building upon a given enabling technology, ultimately, one or several will be widely adopted and others will be discarded.

Since some surgeons are technologically savvy and relish new technology, they are often early adopters, at times making the process of acceptance rapid and underpinning a strong phase of expansion. On the other hand, since many surgeons tend to be risk-averse, long periods of avoidance of change may be seen.

New nomenclature in surgical innovation should focus on recognizing the clinical impact of novel technology, more than market impact. It should also characterize the ebb and flow of technology along a continuum and describe such phases of innovation.

An expanding period of innovation can be defined as a time when technology develops rapidly and patient care is significantly altered. Most enabling technologies and enabling procedures support a network of new technology development and fall within expanding periods.

A refining period of innovation can be defined as a time when existing technologies are improved upon, but patient care is changed little by these improvements. A refining innovation generally either increases efficiency, lessens the labor or device costs for a procedure, or slightly improves outcome. Most disruptive technologies are refining in that they use or improve upon an existing technology while reducing unit cost. Incremental technologies also fit within the category of refining. The terms expanding and refining periods are independent of industry leaders, reflecting historical context and the overall impact of an innovation on patients and providers. It is our opinion that both phases and types of innovation should be recognized as important.

Much of the information presented thus far views innovation as it are described from a business perspective. To further understand each of these concepts as they are applied to the field of surgery, examine the history of surgical endoscopy can tell much. Rather than attempting to describe all important innovations leading to surgical endoscopy, critical elements of its history can be used as a reference to elucidate concepts in innovation.

Since most surgical specialties contributed to advances in surgical endoscopy, the focus will be on surgical innovation as a whole rather than specific subspecialties.

It should be noted that within the history of surgical endoscopy, many aspects are considered great successes while others have been called failures.

The history of endoscopic surgery has been described in multiple phases, generally categorized by progress in underlying technologies: light sources, flexible instruments, and interventional tools. These attributes were developed in parallel and have been well described.

Watching the development of endoscopy could find important elements from the past. But are the last decades of the last century that we want to focus.

By the 1970s and 1980s, a new period of surgical endoscopy expansion had begun. Modern minimal access surgery was largely ushered in through arthroscopy for orthopedics and laparoscopy for gynecologic surgery.

To illustrate fundamental concepts in innovation, an advance in surgical endoscopy which has been exceedingly well documented, the laparoscopic cholecystectomy, is a good example to be examined.

While a relatively late development in surgical endoscopy, the advent of laparoscopic cholecystectomy represented an inflection point for interventional technique and propelled an expanding period of procedural and technologic advancement.

Taking advantage of advances in orthopedic, urologic, and gynecologic technology, Prof Dr Med Erich Mühe of Böblingen, Germany, on September 12, 1985., performed the first laparoscopic cholecystectomy. News of the procedures spread, attracting attention worldwide and leading to rapid research and progress in surgical endoscopy. Newly developed video endoscopy acted as an enabling technology while the operation represented an enabling procedure. The work was disruptive to industry leaders, both corporate and clinical, many of whom initially viewed the process as costly and time- consuming and some of whom were unable to transition to the modern era of laparoscopic intervention. Of note, with disruptive innovation, industry leaders frequently do not recognize the value of a novel technology, providing opportunity to smaller industry firms and individuals.

To assess how innovation occurs, it is necessary to understand individual innovators. Surgeons are fundamentally decision makers. While within most corporations, only top executives make significant leadership decisions, all surgeons face clinical decisions on an hourly basis, many with significant impact and consequence. Furthermore, surgeons in private practice are decision makers within their "firms." Because of necessary frameworks for risk reduction, these individuals are rare within the corporate environment. Based on personality and training, most surgeons leading teams naturally fall within the category of heavyweight. Surgeons have historically been idea generators and creative practitioners within their craft.

In the technology life cycle, the first phase of idea generation and evaluation is fluid and requires vision and flexibility. When asked where the greatest weakness in product innovation is, many managers indicate the idea generation phase. The surgeon's training requires daily situation assessment, decision analysis, and frequent development of new processes. Each clinical case offers unique challenges and requires a degree of creativity. For this reason, surgeons often excel at the creative, fuzzy front end of technology development.

Surgeons understand clinical needs and may anticipate future advances and opportunities. A lead user is defined as a technology user whose present strong needs will become general in a marketplace months or years in the future. Many surgeons are lead users within the field of surgical intervention and instinctively recognize emerging market opportunities. On the other hand, companies often have a difficult time recognizing or competing in emerging markets. Many corporate planning systems do not focus the attention of senior management on unanticipated successes, particularly in new markets. Furthermore, because promotion often depends on short-term accomplishments, managers must distance themselves from the uncertainties inherent in product development while technical personnel protect themselves against the loss of corporate commitment. Because of corporate structure and funding processes, a company's leaders may only be made aware of an emerging market years after a surgeon recognizes the clinical opportunity. This, in part, explains why surgeons have been successful within start up companies in creating disruptive technology. Furthermore, surgeons have the advantage, as thought leaders within a field, to promote a procedure or invention based on clinical outcomes. This practice has come under intense scrutiny with a renewed public and academic focus on conflict of interest. However, it is clear that in the history of surgical innovation, individual proponents of a new process or technology have been essential in its development and adoption.

Although an innovator's personality is critical to new technology development and adoption, context can be just as important. For surgical innovation, we think is fair to use the term context to refer to time and place. The timing of an invention determines not only interest level from the general community, but also technology availability and cost-effectiveness. For an enabling procedure to lead to expansion within a field, the availability of a cluster of new technologies is often required. The place of invention is also surprisingly important. An innovator within a small city is far less likely to have the intellectual interaction and academic connections necessary to have his or her invention noticed. While time may determine technology availability, place will often determine financial and intellectual resources. The externalities, or synergistic benefits associated with location, product adoption, and personal network, are increasingly being recognized.

As an example, history shows how personality and the right context combined to support Mühe as stunningly effective innovator, in developing new technology and bringing it to practice. The proper context currently exist for rapid expansion in nanotechnology, regenerative medicine, and robotics. With the context in place, these fields require effective clinical innovators to bring about new therapies and improved patient care.

While it is clear that surgeons throughout history have acted as innovators critical to the development of new technology and procedures, many innovators find their actions ineffective in influencing the surgical community. Health care has been described as the most entrenched, change-averse industry in the world. Within health care, surgical culture is often seen to be particularly traditional, overly emphasizing our past. It is understandable that the overall tone would be conservative within a field where a radical or novel approach can translate to significant morbidity or mortality.

Still, countless opportunities may be lost as innovators and innovations are ignored or actively rejected by consensus within our field.

While it is clear that the surgeon innovator's personal characteristics are critical to technology development and diffusion, context is equally important. Included in context is community support for surgical innovation.

There are countless historical examples of the surgical community's reluctance to accept change.

As eloquently described by scientific documents in different periods, "new surgical procedures must be tested, and that means clinical testing by mortality and morbidity, and psychologic and social testing by outcome for the individual patient and the community." It may also be noted that laparoscopic cholecystectomy was not evaluated initially by randomized controlled trials but was propelled by anecdotes and case series.

Nevertheless, for a field that is proud of its innovative roots, and in fact, dependent upon them, we often are stingy in our praise for novel ideas and procedures.

It is clear that personal characteristics of the innovator and acceptance of the surgical community are just as critical to innovation as technology and technique. Both enabling and incremental technology changes are important, but both require a fertile ground within which they can take root.

Using the history of surgical endoscopy as a guide, fundamental concepts in technology innovation as they apply to surgery can be examined.

Several new concepts and terms unique to innovation within surgery are also been introduced. While surgical endoscopy reflects only a small subset of innovation within surgery, it is representative of the larger picture. Most will find applicability of these concepts and terms to other stories or personal experiences in innovation.

As a specialty, is just now beginning to analyze and understand what has made some group of researchers the leaders in medical device innovation for the last 2 millennia and which elements have hindered their progress. The current potential for advancement in therapeutic intervention is only rivaled by the mid-1800s with the advent of anesthesia and antisepsis. Rapid advances in imaging, minimally invasive technique, and robotic technology suggest we are at a threshold for a new era in patient care.

There has never been more capital applied to medical technology and devices or more interest in surgical technology development. The successful surgeon innovator of today clearly must be savvy not only in medicine, but also in technology and business. As we continue to draw bright, hard-working, and talented individuals to our ranks, this is well within our grasp.

As a field, we have generated some of the leading innovators in history. We have also discouraged and rejected critical innovations. During this era of unprecedented opportunity and formidable roadblocks, it is time we as a profession take an active role in promoting innovation. In this effort, we must understand historical advances, recognize our successes and mistakes, clarify current challenges and resources, and work to promote a supportive environment within our field. If not us, then who else will take this role? We think that our future depends upon a clear understanding of innovation and rational and strong support of innovators within our specialty.

Chapter 4

What is Smit Map doing?

As it is clear from a careful look at the history of surgical innovation and a deep study of the current state of surgical research, we can see that is absolutely necessary to establish networks of cooperation that can contribute together to have real and enforceable results.

Especially looking at the fact that almost all the research and application centers of innovations in medicine are or, are gradually getting over-specialized and becoming experts in narrow fields of innovative action. We will bring below some examples of how to search and carry out an innovative surgical project is necessary to combine with the professionalism and experience of a considerable number of research centers.

There is another important aspect to consider today; the great opportunity that provides the electronic network. Through which you can involve with excellent results even for individuals or organizations that location would be prevented from expressing their ideas and experience and their potential technological development. Especially at this point and on broad comparisons of professional actors in the field we believe SMIT MAP can play a key role as a network of excellence for technological innovations applied to medicine, particularly in surgery.

Indeed SMIT MAP is already doing this role, and on the work we are presenting, one of the goals is to stress the importance and to study ways to more development of this network.

Now, as already mentioned in previous chapters in SMIT MAP joined many centers, mostly members of SMIT. Some of these centers have a long and laudable history of collaboration in surgical research. The work results of some of these centers is well known and documented in authoritative scientific medical and surgical papers. We can also find descriptions of their work, their fields of activity and specialties browsing through the web site of SMIT MAP. We think this is a good way to search for partnerships when we have a idea to implement.

We think that in this context the same SMIT MAP acts as a true platform connecting centers of excellence through which, can be carried out innovative research in medicine. The confluence on the same platform of centers with different field of experience and action research, creates conditions to have excellent results. The presence of clinical and pre clinical centers, where research results can be tested and validated increases greatly the chances of success of studies carried out.

We proceed by describing the way some vast research projects are organized, by putting together a consortium of companies and academic research centers working on one or more objectives.

We believe that bringing the attention of the initial projects with which started those programs can be the best way to illustrate what our network have and what we want to generate extending the SMIT MAP activity. The choice of these examples, with a surgical basic guidance, already mentioned, in this study, was guided by well known scientific activity of the participants and from the complexity of their projects.

The firs one, VECTOR, "Versatile Endoscopic Capsule for gastrointestinal Tumor Recognition and therapy", arises from the initial idea and collaboration built into Smit Map, by some members that using the platform have design their research project. By Smit Map they sought and found the other research centers to create the necessary joint consortium to give a complete profile and feasible study.

Novineon Healthcare Technology Partners GmbH, Germany, Scuola Superiore Sant' Anna, Italy; Foundation for Scientific and Industrial Research at the Norwegian Institute of Technology, Norway; Endosmart GmbH, Germany; Ovesco Endoscopy AG, Germany; ERA Endoscopy Srl, Italy; Innovent Technology e.V., Germany; are all the members of the Smit Map working in VECTOR. But a fundamental role in the project is served by the same SMIT as one of the parts of the consortium, who, with his authoritative presence as a scientific landmark, helps also in the experimental realization stages of pre- clinical and clinical trials, that are absolutely necessary for the validation of the product. Only after a serious work of validation it is possible to bring the product to its final use. SMIT also, as we can see below, makes an important role in training, dissemination and exploitation which are basic requirements for a successful final result.

The other project we will take as an example, Araknes, that aims at bringing inside the patient's stomach a set of advanced bio-robotic and microsystem technologies for therapy and surgery. It is not a Smit Map project but, our platform though indirectly has a role on the Araknes design. Two of the participants (Novineon Healthcare Technology Partners GmbH, Germany, Scuola Superiore Sant' Anna, Italy) of the consortium of which one also coordinator of the project are as full members of Smit Map. Their fundamental importance in leadership and research roles we believe have much influenced in the creation and implementation of work.

VECTOR
"Versatile Endoscopic Capsule for gastrointestinal Tumor Recognition and therapy"

VECTOR project aims at investigating and developing a miniaturised robotic pill for advanced diagnostics and therapy in the human digestive tract making a significant contribution to the diagnosis and treatment of digestive cancers and their precursors and to strengthen the competitiveness of the European biomedical industry through innovative technologies.

Considering that the Gastrointestinal Cancers are a major healthcare challenge around the world. Colon cancer is among the most frequent causes of death and also gastric cancer is a major threat, mainly in some geographic locations of the world. Cancers of the esophagus are progressing since underlying reflux disease is becoming widespread, linked to overweight, stress and dietary habits. Thus gastrointestinal cancers are a very relevant source of personal suffering and also a reason for significant healthcare spending in the healthcare systems of developed countries. Gastrointestinal cancers will lead to death if they remain untreated or lead to the need of major resective surgery or other aggressive treatments if not treated early enough.

Therefore early detection of Gastrointestinal cancer is paramount in the fight against this group of diseases. If detected at an early stage local treatment means, such as locally circumscribed resection, are feasible. The diagnosis at the stage of precursor disease is even more effective since it does not yet represent malignancy, though it may turn into malignant disease. Among these pre-malignant precursors, called precancerosis, are several types of colon polyps with respect to colon cancer of Barret's esophagus, a consequence of long-lasting gastro esophageal reflux disease, with respect to esophageal carcinoma. If the disease is detected at this stage of pre-malignancy, local therapy, such as tissue resection or destruction, can be used to eradicate the disease before malignant transformation and the onset of invasive cancer.

This golden gap between the presence of pre-malignant disease and the beginning of malignant transformation is typical for several types of Gastrointestinal cancers. This is the key for the medical strategy of early detection and therapy.

That enables and necessitates a global approach by companies, nongovernmental organizations and international bodies to challenge Gastrointestinal cancers.

Early detection programs with screening colonoscopy are widely supported by the medical community and also become integrated into the reimbursement scheme in many countries. However only a fraction of patients make use of screening endoscopy since current procedures can be associated with discomfort and pain. Thus the development of novel painless endoscopic devices is needed to increase cancer screening rates. Wireless capsule endoscopy might be an answer to this problem, but current passive capsules cannot replace conventional endoscopy in terms of diagnostic and therapeutic performance. Advanced technology can enhance capsule endoscopy to a level at which it can compete with traditional endoscopy. This development is the medical background of the VECTOR project.

There are still major limitations to the technologies and procedures available for endoscopically detecting and treating GI cancers. Among the key problems are the design of the flexible endoscope itself and the method endoscopy is done today. The limited flexibility of the endoscope combined with the pushing techniques applied today for advancing the device into the human body is associated with procedural pain, limiting the willingness of the patients to undergo endoscopic procedures, especially for screening purposes. Propulsion or locomotion technologies to overcome the classical scheme of endoscopy, without the need of artificially pushing an endoscope through the digestive tract will therefore be of paramount importance for increasing patient compliance and screening rates.

Other restrictions in the field of endoscopic diagnosis are limited tissue analysis capabilities to improve tumour detection. New developments in the field of sensors and optical techniques allow helping with the detection of characteristic features of tumour cells and tissues.

Finally, improved treatment capabilities for tissue resection and destruction or the local application of drugs will be required to combine enhanced diagnostic with therapeutic functions.

Considering those technological concepts was important for the project designers to extend an accurate work program involving a large number of components/collaborators inside.

The project is a multi disciplinary, cross-sectorial technology development project at the crossroads on one side between technology and medicine and science and business on the other side. Therefore the management structure of the project needs to reflect the interdisciplinary nature of the programme. Considering the VECTOR system as a minirobot endowed with actuation modules, mechanisms, sensors, embedded control and human-machine interface, and with the challenging task to navigate in and intervene in to the gastrointestinal tract, the work was divided into several work packages. To any of them was selected a Work Package leader, other components interested on the field and obviously a specific objective and relative time lines to proceed.

We will describe the different package and the relative objective of work.

- **Project Management:**

Who's objective is to provide management capacities to the project and to ensure proper organization and management of the consortium. On that participate *all the consortium components.*

- **Medical and Technological Background & System Requirements:** *Participants: Novineon Healthcare Technology Partners GmbH, Germany (leader WP), SSSA Scuola Superiore Sant' Anna, Italy, SINTEF Foundation for Scientific and Industrial Research at the Norwegian Institute of Technology (NTH), Norway, KU-Leuven, Belgium, EPFL Ecole Polytechnique Fédérale de Lausanne, Switzerland, CTMN Centre de transfert en micro & nanotechnologies, France, SMIT Society for Medical Innovation and Technology e.V. International and Innovent Technology e.V., Germany*

This work package will study the medical and technological background in order to define the VECTOR system requirements.

In particular, the medical requirements of smart capsules for cancer diagnosis and treatment in the gastrointestinal tract would include biomedical parameters for locomotion, tissue properties for diagnosis and concepts for treatment.

An in depth technology analysis will cover all aspects related to the technology platforms that are eligible to meet the goals of the project and to realize the medical requirements for smart GI capsules. The main objective of the technology review is to highlight those solutions with the potential to be introduced in the smart capsule without wasting resources in developing ad hoc technologies for each specific task. Being VECTOR a very multidisciplinary and multi-sectorial project, the technological background requires competences ranging from biomedical engineering, to electronic engineering, mechanical engineering, information science and physics. In addition, it is crucial that the medical background and the technological background proceed in parallel, in order to focus always and only on the technologies which are useful for the specific medical problems addressed by VECTOR.

Both medical and technological background will form the basis to formulate the user requirements for the developments within VECTOR.

- **Market & Regulatory Framework:**

Participants: Novineon Healthcare Technology Partners GmbH, Germany (leader WP), *KIST Europe GmbH, Germany, ERA Endoscopy Srl, Italy, SMIT Society for Medical Innovation and Technology e.V., Germany, netMED AISBL, Belgium* and *Innovent Technology e.V., Germany*

- **Health-Economic Impact & Outcomes Analysis:**

Participants: Novineon Healthcare Technology Partners GmbH, Germany (leader WP) and SSSA Scuola Superiore Sant' Anna, Italy

The health-economic impact is an important parameter to qualify the medical feasibility of technology. This is mainly based on the analysis of medical outcomes and the monetary resources involved into realizing these outcomes. Therefore the consortium will dedicate a work package to this item in order to demonstrate the benefits of smart capsules for healthcare systems. The work package partly uses results created in work package 2 but is clearly separate from this work package. The purpose of the second work package is to analyse the health-economic outcome of the VECTOR devices as a justification for future clinical use. This kind of outcome analysis requires concrete input and substantial knowledge about the factual performance of the devices and procedures to be studied.

- **Design and Dimensioning of the Robotic Pill / Platform and its Variations:**

Partecipants: SSSA Scuola Superiore Sant' Anna, Italy (leader WP), Sensitec GmbH, Germany, KU Leuven, Belgium, CTMN Centre de transfert en micro & nanotechnologies, France, Endosmart GmbH, Germany, University of Barcelona, Spain, FORTH Foundation for research and technologies Hellas, Greece, Innovent Technology e.V., Germany, Jagiellonian University, Poland and NeuriCam SPA, Italy

This work package will take care of aligning the numerous technical parameters related to the smart capsule, such as power consumption, compatibility issues, basic functions and all related constraints. The main result is a modular architecture of the smart capsule system for the development of preliminary and advanced prototypes. This architecture will consider both the main modules of the capsule (vision, locomotion, telemetry, power) and the modular parts, which could be different depending on the different diagnosis and therapy procedures which will be selected.

- **Locomotion & Space Creation:**

Participants: SSSA Scuola Superiore Sant' Anna, Italy (leader WP), Novineon Healthcare Technology Partners GmbH, Germany, Sensitec GmbH, Germany, KU Leuven, Belgium, CTMN Centre de transfert en micro & nanotechnologies, France, Endosmart GmbH, Germany, ERA Endoscopy Srl, Italy, University of Barcelona, Spain, FORTH Foundation for research and technologies Hellas, Greece, Innovent Technology e.V., Germany and IMC Intelligent Microsystem Center, South Korea

This work package aims at studying, model, and develop an active locomotion system for the smart capsule. Active locomotion is one of the most important key features of the capsule, because it allows performing controlled diagnosis and therapy in selected areas of the gut. Active systems for space creation are also essential to distend the tissues for proper diagnosis and visualization, and to create a real lumen which, otherwise, is just virtual.

Commercially available digestive capsules rely on peristaltic locomotion [e.g. Given Imaging] or on external system of orientation (Norika, Olympus), which do not possess adequate flexibility for locomotion in tortuous environment. Moreover, no available systems include active space creation mechanism, thus limiting the effectiveness in selected areas of the gut (the small intestine). Based on the above considerations, an active locomotion system allowing the capsule to move independently from peristalsis and a mechanism for space creation stem mainly from a medical need are under investigation. The most promising solution, especially for the colon district, seems to be the "legged" locomotion. As regards space creation, balloons or enlarging structures are arguments under investigation.

- **Vision System & Illumination:**

44

Participants: SSSA Scuola Superiore Sant' Anna, Italy (leader WP), EPFL Ecole Polytechnique Fédérale de Lausanne, Switzerland, Endosmart GmbH, Germany, University of Barcelona, Spain, FORTH Foundation for research and technologies Hellas, Greece, IMC Intelligent Microsystem Center, South Korea, Jagiellonian University, Poland and NeuriCam SPA, Italy

Vision is one of the key elements for endoscopic diagnosis. The challenge of the R&D for the vision and illumination system is realizing a very compact, high performance and low power imaging system. This will require a very efficient illumination system and a very sensitive camera. In order to achieve this goal all components have to be optimized and tuned to each other. Besides the power management, the thermal management will be a specific issue. Strategies for color reconstruction, autofocus and zoom functions have to be developed and implemented. The maximum data rate, a product of resolution and frame rate, has to be considered and probably data compression strategies will be important. Other areas of concern are auto exposure control and high dynamic range handling strategies. A clear vision has also to be maintained during time, thus making mandatory a vision maintenance system (e.g. lens cleaning system).

- **Integrated Circuit Development:**

Participants: University of Barcelona, Spain (leader WP) and SSSA Scuola Superiore Sant' Anna, Italy

Taking into account the very small dimensions of the capsule, full custom Integrated Circuits have to be designed and implemented to properly drive and control the robotic device. Low voltage integrated circuits will be developed in order to increase the integration level and minimize the final circuit surface. High yield in power conversion is a big challenge due to the small amount of energy available in the capsule. The energy capacity limitation of the power source will call for power recovery techniques, used to increase the robot autonomy. High density assembling and packaging techniques have to be combined to adapt the electronic modules to the capsule. Different functions will be defined to drive walking mechanisms, to acquire and elaborate signals from the frontal camera, to send and receive signals through the telemetric link, and to operate the diagnostic and therapeutic units. Close co-operation with the other work packages will ensure a final size and performances optimization. A control strategy for the motion drives will be implemented. Some intelligence has to be included to overcome non-linear behaviour of the actuation system in order to increase the accuracy of motion. Power circuitry and digital control system have to be integrated in a mixed mode Integrated Circuits along with sensor read-out circuits and signal communication transceivers. By using multi chip packaging, "on board" electronics could be included: power step up conversion, power signal generation, IR (or RF) driving circuitry, IR (or RF) interface protocol, etc. The full custom Integrated Circuits for the main body of the capsule will include all the electronic interfaces with the capsule's sub modules. Moreover several Integrated Circuits for the different derivative device will be designed in order to enable the autonomous operation of each one of them.

- **Sensors for Diagnosis:**

Participants: EPFL Ecole Polytechnique Fédérale de Lausanne, Switzerland (leader WP), SINTEF Foundation for Scientific and Industrial Research at the Norwegian Institute of Technology (NTH), Norway, CTMN Centre de transfert en micro & nanotechnologies, France, University of Barcelona, Spain and NeuriCam SPA, Italy

Sensor enhancements are critical in order to achieve disruptive diagnostic performances in the field of capsular endoscopy. These performances include optical sensor functions, such as fluorescence and diffused light spectroscopy, ultrasound transducers to assess tissue properties like inflammation (as well as for navigation), mechanical sensors to assess biomechanical tissue properties, as well as biochemical sensors or biosensors to identify tumour specific substances. Very important parameters for advanced diagnostics are pressure (to verify the peristaltic work of the intestine), pH (to evaluate the chemical content of the intestine) and temperature sensors. The work package includes the development and integration of a set of passive sensors for the measurement of these parameters, based on the principle of a remote interrogation (no need of any power supply) in a frequency domain of 433 or 866 MHz.

- **Tissue Sampling & Treatment:**

Participants: Endosmart GmbH, Germany (leader WP),Novineon Healthcare Technology Partners GmbH, Germany, KIST Europe GmbH, Germany, CTMN Centre de transfert en micro & nanotechnologies, France, Ovesco Endoscopy AG, Germany and Innovent Technology e.V., Germany

Sampling of cells and tissues is a relevant step in the diagnosis of cancer. Therefore tissue sampling means are important for the concept of intelligent capsules for the gastrointestinal tract. The treatment functions of the capsule are closely associated to the tissue sampling, since this will involve mechanical tissue removal techniques. Besides these mechanical functions, also thermal tissue destruction techniques as well as the release of fluids, such as locally acting drugs will be investigated. It is the objective that this will involve advanced pharmaceutical tumour treatment concepts, such as antibody therapy.

- **Power Supply:**

Participants: SSSA Scuola Superiore Sant' Anna, Italy (leader WP), KU Leuven, Belgium and Endosmart GmbH, Germany

Who's aim is to develop means for the electrical powering of the smart capsule. In fact all the tasks, which have to be performed by the device while operating inside the human body (locomotion, tissue sampling, drug delivery, communication, etc), require a substantial amount of energy which no off-the shelf products are able to provide, so that tailored solutions have to be investigated and developed. Hybrid powering strategies, such as wireless power transmission and power storage, are actually under investigation.

- **Navigation & Localization:**

Participants: Innovent Technology e.V., Germany (leader WP), SSSA Scuola Superiore Sant' Anna, Italy, SINTEF Foundation for Scientific and Industrial Research at the Norwegian Institute of Technology (NTH), Norway, Sensitec GmbH, Germany, CTMN Centre de transfert en micro & nanotechnologies, France, FORTH

Foundation for research and technologies Hellas, Greece and Jagiellonian University, Poland

Diagnosis and therapeutic interventions require precise and reliable navigation and localization. The objective is to construct in collaboration with other work packages an accurate system for remote navigation and localization of the device. Navigation of the smart capsule in reference to prior capsule investigation collected external diagnostic imaging, such as CT or MRI image data sets, is an important medical demand. Therefore an individual work package is devoted to this particular topic. Additional efforts will be devoted to investigate the best suited localization techniques that do not rely on radiological imaging, such as (electro-)magnetic localizers, inertial sensors and vision-based localization.

The objective is a capsule that can be localized without having a radiological imaging examination. Therefore magnetic localization is favored.

• **Communication & Telemetry Issues:**

Participants: KU Leuven, Belgium (leader WP) and Jagiellonian University, Poland

The endoscopic capsule needs also a bidirectional data transmission for its operation. The downlink from the capsule to the outside world must be able to transmit a large amount of data. The available data rate will define the image quality of the endoscope. However, to get a high data rate one needs to increase the radio frequency of the carrier wave of the signal; but the higher the frequency, the higher the absorption of the waves by the human body. As the available power for the transmission is limited, a dedicated transmitter will be needed. The definition of the protocol is also part of the radio transmission since it will affect the Bit Error Rate of the system.

The uplink, from outside the body to the capsule, does not need a high data rate since the only commands are transmitted through this link. However it needs to be highly secured to avoid any unexpected comportment of the capsule while travelling through the human body. Therefore the protocol must be extremely robust in order to let the physician rely on it.

• **Control System & User Interface:**

Participants: FORTH Foundation for research and technologies Hellas, Greece (leader WP) and SSSA Scuola Superiore Sant' Anna, Italy

The group of this work package is concentrated in the design, modelling and implementation of motion control for the capsule, aiming both at the generation of open-loop gaits in the challenging locomotion environment of the GI tract, and at the generation of sensor-driven closed-loop reactive behaviours, necessary in order to endow the capsule with some limited navigational autonomy. The main control goals are efficient locomotion of the pill and the avoidance of damages to the delicate GI tissues. Moreover, this WP will address the development of an easy and intuitive user interface, which will be used to control the capsule.

- **System Integration of the Prototype:**

Participants: SSSA Scuola Superiore Sant' Anna, Italy (leader WP), Endosmart GmbH, Germany and IMC Intelligent Microsystem Center, South Korea

After the optimization of all components of the system, the integration phase is very delicate and critical. The system integration represents the connection between technology and medical application. The assembly of every biomedical instrumentation requires the knowledge of all mechanical, electrical, thermal and biological interfaces. All the medical constraints (safety issues, biocompatibility etc.) will be considered in this phase. As soon as the consortium defines the main features of the sub-modules, an accurate investigation about the best solutions for the integration and packaging will be carried out. This investigation will be based on the choice of the external material, glues, assembly technologies, biological interfaces, etc. The system integration phase must not be necessarily limited to the final part of the project: the development of preliminary prototypes will help to define the system- integration process step by step. Medical certification aspects, e.g. final risk management, will be taken into account at this step of the project as, after assembling the pre clinical and clinical trial, it can be prepared only after receiving the necessary certifications regarding the guidelines.

- **Medical Assessment, Pre-Clinical & Clinical Studies**:

Participants Novineon Healthcare Technology Partners GmbH, Germany (leader WP), SINTEF Foundation for Scientific and Industrial Research at the Norwegian Institute of Technology (NTH), Norway and SMIT Society for Medical Innovation and Technology e.V., Germany

The medical assessment of the technologies and devices created will be an ongoing effort and involve not only the assessment of the final prototypes but also of the interim steps and of the derivative device developed on the pathway.

The objective of the work package on medical assessment is to provide direct medical feedback to those consortium partners engaged with technology development. This is not only important at the end of the project for the final validation of prototypes but also during the course of development in order to ensure technologies are developed according to medical requirements and the preconditions.

- **Derivatives & Spin-off Devices**:

Participants: Ovesco Endoscopy AG, Germany (leader WP), Endosmart GmbH, Germany, ERA Endoscopy Srl, Italy, University of Barcelona, Spain and FORTH Foundation for research and technologies Hellas, Greece

In order to ensure a proper transfer of the technology developed within the scope of the VECTOR project into future products, the project partners will work on derivative solutions of the smart capsule technology that can be employed into medical use during the pathway of the research program. For this purpose, the technology platforms of the smart capsule, e.g. those for locomotion, tissue manipulation, or tumor recognition, will be assessed according to their suitability, usability, requirements for immediate medical use, and medical indications by means of prototypes of derivative devices.

The derivative devices will be adapted to currently used medical procedures and methods, in order to obtain information about the said aspects, taking into account the medical reality. This process enables specific functions of the technology platforms for the smart capsule to be tested and verified in the medical world before the complete smart capsule system is available.

This information supports the project partners to continuously orientate the development process to the basic requirements by learning from the experiences collected with derivative devices. Thus, the work within the scope of the work package 15 serves as a constructive feedback mechanism and guideline to enable the project partners to optimize research pathway, apart from its genuine function to make VECTOR technology platforms available for medical use as soon as possible.

A further objective of the work package is to maximize the exploitation of the R&D results by adapting derivative devices to neighbouring medical applications. For this purpose, individual results of the development work are verified for medical usability by means of experimental prototypes of the respective derivative device. With this early technology transfer approach, the project partners are aiming at exploiting the R&D results for non-capsule applications as well. This also supports the communication with the clinical community through making derivative devices practically available among the users; thus the future medical introduction of smart capsules will be easier thanks to these technology platforms.

- **Training, Dissemination and Exploitation:**

Participants: netMED AISBL, Belgium (leader WP), Novineon Healthcare Technology Partners GmbH, Germany, SSSA Scuola Superiore Sant' Anna, Italy and SMIT Society for Medical Innovation and Technology e.V., Germany Dissemination of research results, training and exploitation will be actively pursued by the consortium. These activities are led by a company, that holds a significant expertise in medical dissemination, training and exploitation.

All the results, both research, state of the art and market analysis will be disseminated first among the partners of the consortium and then to the scientific community through specialized media, as selected magazines, conferences, fairs, web sites. This will contribute to make known the competences of the consortium and the results of VECTOR through the medical society, including clinicians considered final users and patients, through the biomedical and micro engineering companies, through the technologists i.e. Engineering Faculties etc.

Training activities will be carried out based on the dissemination activities, the target of the courses is expected essentially coming from the medical community, the Engineering universities and highly specialized biomedical companies.

As we can se the goal of the project is to enable medical devices through advanced technology that can dramatically improve early detection and treatment of gastrointestinal early cancers and cancer precursors projecting innovative microsystems components, micro-robotic technologies and sensor devices for novel applications in this medical field and to provide groundbreaking technology leads and platform technologies to European biomedical companies for future conversion into competitive novel products. This shall support the European biomedical industry in the international medical device market and help build up a franchise in the booming sector of cancer prevention, early diagnosis and treatment technologies.

ARAKNES

"Array of Robots Augmenting the Kinematics of Endoluminal Surgery" The system that ARAKNES program propose, advances the current endoscopic surgical procedures by adding the bi-manual tele-operation equivalent to that of laparoscopic surgical robots integrating the advantages of traditional open surgery, laparoscopic surgery and robotics surgery into a deeply innovative system for bi-manual, ambulatory, tethered, visible scarless surgery, based on an array of smart microrobotic instrumentation.

In traditional open surgery, physical and rigid links exist between the surgeon and the patient's organs. The instruments are hand-held and operated under direct binocular vision.

With the introduction of laparoscopic techniques, the direct physical links between the surgeon and the patient's organs are represented by the trocars, which are used for the insertion of different instruments, energised dissection devices and staplers all having a remote end-effector and proximal actuation i.e., the surgeon's hand

Surgical tele-operated robots are considered an important on-going evolution in minimally invasive surgery because whilst the main features of surgical execution are retained, the actuation of bi-manual tools is remote from the patient and is performed by the surgeon operating from a console.

Finally, in flexible interventional endoscopy, the rigid link between the surgeon and the organs becomes progressively weaker as the mechanical constraints are transferred from outside the body to lumen of an internal hollow organ. Mechanically as exemplified by the autonomous colonoscopes, the rigid transmission from outside is removed.

The medical background of that program is locking to work on interventions for morbid obesity and gastroesophageal reflux disease.

The components that underpin ARAKNES emphasises the development of new surgical technology based on the "Micro/nano/bio convergence". The development of the robotic platform will go in parallel with the development of its teleoperation control system and the dedicated human machine interface. All MEMS, NEMS, sensing devices and lab-on-chip components will be specifically developed by the different partners or will be adapted from other fields covered by the ARAKNES Consortium. The team of clinicians will be also responsible for the medical assessment of the project results in conjunction with companies specialising in medical device validation.

Based on the outlined general strategy, has been organized a work plan what we are going to describe.

Were selected 11 packages, engaging between the components of the consortium one leader and other research centres in each work packages. Working in **medical and technological background** the selected group (*Novineon Healthcare Technology Partners GmbH, Germany (leader WP),Scuola Superiore Sant' Anna, Pisa, Italy, Imperial College of London, University of Pisa, Italy; Ecole Polytechnique Fédérale de Lausanne, Switzerland; Microtech Srl., Italy; Karl Storz Gmbh & Co, Germany; St Microelectronics, Italy; The University Court of the University of St Andrews, UK; University of Barcelona, Spain; Laboratory of*

Computer Sciences and Robotics and Microelcetronics, France) will study the medical and technological background in order to define the ARAKNES system requirements. An in-depth technology analysis will cover all aspects related to the technology platforms that are eligible to meet the goals of the project and to realize the medical requirements for the gastric surgical platform.

The main objective of the technology review is to highlight those solutions with the potential to be introduced in the platform without wasting resources in developing ad hoc technologies for each specific task. ARAKNES being a very multidisciplinary and multi-sectorial project, the technological background requires competences ranging from biomedical engineering, to electronic engineering, mechanical engineering, information science and physics.

Giving particular emphasis to Intellectual Property Right (IPR) search, in order to understand and direct the development of novel devices toward market exploitation of results. In addition considering crucial that the medical background and the technological background proceed in parallel, in order to focus always and only on the technologies which are useful for the specific medical problems addressed by the program objectives.

Starting from the medical and technological background relevant to the ARAKNES objectives and assessed in **surgical method and system architecture**, (*Novineon Healthcare Technology Partners GmbH, Germany (leader WP),_Scuola Superiore Sant' Anna, Pisa, Italy, Imperial College of London, University of Pisa, Italy; Ecole Polytechnique Fédérale de Lausanne, Switzerland The University Court of the University of St Andrews, UK; University of Barcelona, Spain; Laboratory of Computer Sciences and Robotics and Microelcetronics, France)* innovative surgical procedures are defined by the medical partners of the project. In the frame of this work package a close collaboration between the medical and the technological partners is of utmost importance. The main outcomes will be the description of the targeted procedures to be achieved using the ARAKNES platform and a detailed system architecture, where all the possible interfaces among the different modules are clearly identified.

The group working on **assistive and operative platform** (*Ecole Polytechnique Fédérale de Lausanne Switzerland (leader WP), Scuola Superiore Sant' Anna, Pisa, Italy ; Microtech Srl., Italy*) has the objective to develop the ARAKNES operative room in the gastric endoluminal site, by accessing it through a dedicated insertion port, by creating the required space and by developing robotic modular units capable of displacement and onboard arm motion and by developing the endoluminal robotic frames, that will serve as mechanical references of the micro robots, having safe deployment, refolding and retrieval capability. This includes defining the hardware and software interfaces to guarantee the compatibility between the platform subsystems and overall platform integration.

To develop innovative devices for endoluminal monitoring and therapy, that can be integrated on the miniature manipulators of the endoluminal robotic modules. Three different kinds of devices will be addressed in **Micro and Nano Systems for endoluminal monitoring and therapy** work package(*University of Barcelona, Spain (leader WP),Scuola Superiore Sant'Anna, Pisa, Italy; Karl Storz Gmbh & Co, Germany; Stm Microelectronics, Italy; The University Court of the University of St Andrews, UK Laboratory of Computer Sciences and Robotics*).

The development of multi-sensors based on polymeric technology for real-time monitoring of pH, blood gases, electrolytes, and some selected metabolites, especially when such compounds are subject to a rapid change inside the body (Development of multi-sensors based on silicon technologies), Lab-on-a-chip based on microfluidics and spectroscopic analyses (Optics & Photonics based technologies for in situ monitoring, diagnostics and therapy), MEMS based micro devices (Microtechnologies and MEMS for Endoluminal End- Effectors).

Mostly the adaptation of existing devices to the ARAKNES endoluminal platform will be pursued, with particular emphasis on smart system integration, miniaturization and packaging. Design of novel devices will also be considered, especially to cover particular medical needs that may arise from the second and third work package. Wireless operation of the single devices will also be studied once the tethered versions will be validated and assessed. The **Optical**

System Development (*Karl Storz Gmbh & Co, Germany (leader WP),Scuola Superiore Sant' Anna, Pisa, Italy*; *The University Court of the University of St Andrews, UK)* objective is the generation of a concept and a model of a micro-imaging device including illumination and vision, based on semiconductor technology. To meet these objectives, a multi-element vision system will be designed and evaluated. Imaging modules for frontal but also side-viewing capabilities are necessary. Due to the limited size of the delivery device (that is basically the oro-pharyngo- esophageal-access port) a lateral oriented robot with side view imaging and lateral oriented tools seem to be essential to fulfil the requirements of the endoluminal application.

Based on the key concept of array of micro-robots, the proposed system in the ARAKNES project has to be controlled in order to provide the surgeon with the expected capabilities at just the right time depending on the task he has to perform. Therefore, beyond the mandatory real-time operating control architecture of the tethered system and the definition control modes, the objectives of **Teleoperation and Robot control** work package(*Laboratory of Computer Sciences and Robotics and Microelcetronics, France (leader WP),Scuola Superiore Sant' Anna, Pisa, Italy; Imperial College of London, University of Pisa, Italy; Ecole Polytechnique Fédérale de Lausanne, Switzerland)* concerns the development of a control architecture dedicated to the control of an array of micro-robots including a bimanual and bilateral scheme with force feedback. It should ensure stability and transparency with respect to the heterogeneous environment, thus providing the surgeon with a good feedback of the various interactions between the robots and the tissues. Finally the whole system should comply with the long-term wireless constraints.

The **Console** work package(*Imperial College of London (leader WP), University of Pisa, Italy; Ecole Polytechnique Fédérale de Lausanne, Switzerland; Karl Storz Gmbh & Co, Germany)* working to develop the perceptual docking platform to enhance the surgeon's interaction with the robot and provide effective control, guidance and visualization throughout the real or simulated interventional procedure. To meet this objective, the package is divided into the following aims:

• Provide a console based image guidance system with augmented reality visualization making use of real-time 3D information recovered optically from the operating field in conjunction with preoperative and intraoperative medical imaging data.

• Integrate perceptual docking on the master console by using eye tracking information to give surgeon a unique way of interacting with the robotic system and provide enhanced human-machine synergy.

• Integrate force and haptic feedback on the master controls of console to give the surgeon a sense of touch as well as enforce dynamic active constraints to protect delicate anatomical structures.

Where possible existing technology platforms will be used to meet these tasks. Hardware development is foreseen in: (1) haptics and force feedback device with sensing (2) eye tracking platform. The remainder of the work package will be software focused particularly addressing the development of a video processing capability and the algorithms for meeting the outlined aims and the engineering of an integrated platform for simulation, planning and intraoperative assistance.

To integrate all the modules in a single platform, going from the distal robotic units to the external human machine interface and console is the aim of a specific package also. It includes alto integration of the wireless teleoperation. After the separate testing and optimization of all components of the system, the integration phase is very delicate and critical.

The **system integration** (*Scuola Superiore Sant' Anna, Pisa, Italy (leader WP), Imperial College of London, University of Pisa, Italy; Ecole Polytechnique Fédérale de Lausanne, Switzerland; Karl Storz Gmbh & Co, Germany; University of Barcelona, Spain; Laboratory of Computer Sciences and Robotics and Microelcetronics, France*) represents the connection between technology and medical application. The assembly of every biomedical instrumentation requires the knowledge of all mechanical, electrical, thermal and biological interfaces. All the medical constraints (safety issues, biocompatibility etc.) must be considered in this phase.

This phase must not be necessarily limited to the final part of the project: the development of preliminary prototypes will help to define the system-integration process step by step. Medical certification aspects, e.g. final risk management, have to be taken into account at this step of the project as, after assembling the pre clinical and clinical trial, it can be prepared only after receiving the necessary certifications regarding the guidelines.

The medical assessment of the technologies, systems and devices created will be an ongoing effort and involve not only the assessment of the final prototypes, but also of the interim steps and of the derivative devices developed on the pathway in order to ensure technologies and systems are developed according to medical requirements and the preconditions.

The objectives on medical assessment is to provide direct medical feedback to the Consortium partners engaged with technology development and to provide an evaluation of the safety and functionalities of the ARAKNES platform and all its sub-systems.

Four tasks are focused respectively on the development of experimental test beds and setup, on the assessment of the platform from the point of view of the user and of the patient, and the **medical assessment and experimental validation** (*University of Pisa, Italy (leader WP), Scuola Superiore Sant' Anna, Pisa, Italy, Imperial College of London,; Ecole Polytechnique Fédérale de Lausanne, Switzerland; Microtech Srl., Italy; Laboratory of ComputerSciences and Robotics and Microelcetronics, France and Novineon Healthcare Technology Partners GmbH, Germany)* of the ARAKNES platform prototypes and sub-systems.

Dissemination, Exploitation and Training (*Laboratory of Computer Sciences and Robotics and Microelcetronics, France (leader WP),Scuola Superiore Sant' Anna, Pisa, Italy, Imperial College of London, University of Pisa, Italy; Ecole Polytechnique Fédérale de Lausanne, Switzerland; Microtech Srl., Italy; Karl Storz Gmbh & Co, Germany; St Microelectronics, Italy; The University Court of the University of St Andrews, UK; University of Barcelona, Spain and Novineon Healthcare Technology Partners GmbH, Germany)* is the other package including three complementary and parallel lines of action. Dissemination groups the activities aimed at widely informing about the ARAKNES approach and results, as a condition for their adoption and exploitation in different contexts. A website (www.araknes.org) is developed to deliver information about the project; events are and will be organised and other dissemination activities will be studied and performed. All the partners are somehow engaged in dissemination activities, in particular academic partners to spread the scientific, medical and technological results.

Exploitation groups the activities aimed at establishing the conditions under which the partners participate, in conjunction and separately, in the exploitation of the project results. In particular, plans are made to promote the use of the surgical robotic platform and to commercially exploit any derivative device that can outcome from the project. An Exploitation Agreement will be issued to regulate exploitation rights, special use conditions and relations with third parties. Training activities, addressed both to experts and the general public, organise and promote, teaching material will be prepared by the lecturer and possible locations will be defined according to the partners' competences in the respective area.

As clear on the examples above, the complexity of the fields which impact surgical innovation today determines the need for collaboration of many different specialized centres on different branches, especially in surgery, technology and socioeconomic.

We see that in the program design, was of paramount importance the involvement of shuttle companies specializing in technology research in electronics, chemistry, physics and mechanics. Some members of the consortium are particularly skilled in managing the marketing of the product and others are engaged in the scientific dissemination and training required. Another great importance aspect is given the management of financial resources and above all to find these resources. Of course all them working near clinicians/surgeons.

Another aspect of fundamental importance is the fact that the implementation of research projects designed and conducted by consortia of small and medium enterprises in their modus operandi are not guided by the simple future gains in the marketing of the product. Such a general public or non profit those are substantially supported by public resources and have the possibility to direct more their attention to the needs of the scientific subject of the clinical research. This is not to underestimate the importance of industrial research, we only think that our way is very important because good ideas should not be underestimated for the needs of the market.

Conclusions

Traditional approaches to research and development of medical technology dramatically reduce the potential for innovation and the successful exploitation of scientific discoveries and novel concepts.

Universities, life science companies, clinicians and healthcare providers need to indicate the conduit from lab to clinic. All too often this conduit is blocked by the lack of integration of objectives, plans, operations and funding. Even within universities, the traditional divisions between scientific disciplines (physical sciences, medicine, biology, engineering, etc.) slows down or prevents innovation and successful clinical use. More, the divisions with external stakeholders (clinicians, healthcare providers, life science companies, investors, etc.) can reduce further the impact innovation, implementation and exploitation.

The SMIT MAP is a dedicated tool that integrates a wide range of expertise available across all disciplines and combines it with academic and corporate research partners and investors. All that can bridges the traditional gap between scientific research and the conception and implementation of novel biomedical devices and clinical procedures. The result is unequalled innovation and speed of implementation from lab to clinic.

This Network assemble groups of expert business developers, physicists, engineers, life scientists and clinicians in their focus areas. These groups share and disseminate their research, and brainstorm potentially exciting opportunities for advancing clinical treatments.

This platform is an excellent means of tapping into a powerful network that can:

·   Provide innovative ideas that couldn't be sourced internally

·   Comprehensively evaluate these ideas

·   Provide technical solutions and keep your corporate development teams up-to-speed with the state-of-the-art in multiple areas of research

·   Help inform and direct longer-term, publicly-funded research to enable future innovation of direct value to your business

·   Provide an effective, certified development environment for new technology/products, up to and including pre-clinical trials

Establish and develop links to from the earliest stage in development

·   Help reduce the cost and financial risk of early-stage development by leveraging external funding sources

Smit Map to investors can:

·   Increase their deal flow by providing a pipeline of very well-developed venture opportunities backed by strong IP and comprehensive market research

·   Help their perform clinical and technical due diligence on potential investments

·   De-risk their investments by providing integrated technology or product development services to their investor companies, up to and including pre- clinical trials.

·   De-risk their investments by helping investor companies leverage external (public) funding

However, this is the specific aim of the SMIT Map Network of Excellence program established between founders in the SMIT Conference in 2005.

The only basic requirement to ask to join, is the membership to our prestigious Society, SMIT, that lasts now more than 20 years. The project of the SMIT Map to offer a useful service to help promoting more research in medical technology and innovation, which is our mission.

This research was designed to present and explain SMIT Map as an initial but valuable opportunity of innovative research in medical and surgical field in Europe and more. Today we could not find a suitable program of the European Commission that would support a platform like this. During this research we concluded that in 2010, should there be a call within FP7 program of the Commission, relevant to our type of work, we would be ready to apply.

We very much hope, that this document will clarify the basic importance of a platform that builds a Network of Excellence for innovative research in medicine and surgery and, that may drive those with power to fund this type of work, stand to gain from this, medicine and especially the people. Perhaps we could say, that day, that it had not worked in vain.

At last I really hope SMIT MAP and other similar realities can help to involve on medical generally and surgical innovations specially, researches and birth centres localized in small countries like my own, that working within strict boundaries have little chance to contribute to innovations in medicine.

References

1. Alessandro Laviano, A Network of Excellence, THE LANCET May 8, 2004, Vol 363: 1554.

2.   *Allen S.Lee, Jonathan Liebenau, Janice I. DeGross; Information systems and qualitative research, Chapmann & Hall, 1997*

3.Banta HD. *Minimally Invasive Therapy (MIT) in Five European Countries*. Amsterdam: Elsevier, 1993.

4. Callon, M. (1991): Techno-economic Networks and Irreversibility. In J. Law (ed.): <i>A Sociology of Monsters. Essays on Power, Technology and Domination</i>. Routledge, pp. 132-161.

5. Caplan, A.I. (2000) "Tissue Engineering Designs for the Future: New Logics, Old Molecules" *Tissue Engineering 6, 17-33*

6. Christensen CM, Bohmer R, Kenagy J. Will disruptive innovations cure health care? *Harvard Business Rev.* 2000;78:102–112.

7. Christensen CM. *The Innovator's Dilemma*.New York: HarperCollins, 1997:15–16.

8.Clark K, Wheelwright S. Organizing and leading heavyweight development teams. *Calif Manage Rev.* 1992;34:9–28.

9. Clarke HC. History of endoscopic and laparoscopic surgery. *World J Surg.* 2001;25:967–968.

10. Clarke L, Clarke M, Clarke T. How useful are Cochrane reviews in identifying research needs? Journal of Health Services Research & Policy.2007;12:101–103

11. Clarke M. Doing new research? Don't forget the old. PLoS Medicine. 2004;1:e35.

12. Commission of the European Communities, Communication from the Commission to the Council, the European Parliament, The Economic and social Committee and the Committee of the Regions, Towards a European research area, Brussels, 18.1.2000, COM(2000) 6.

13. Communication from the Commission Competitive European Regions through research and innovation. Brussels, 16.8.2007, COM(2007) 474 final{SEC(2007)1045}.

14. Council of the European Union, Council approves EU research programmes for 2007-2013 Brussels, 18 December 2006, 16887/06 (Press 366)

15. Cooper NJ, Jones DR, Sutton AJ. The use of systematic reviews when designing new studies. Clinical Trials. 2005;2:260–264.

16. Cosgrove DM. The innovation imperative. *J Thorac Cardiovasc Surg.* 2000;120:839–842.

17. *D. Stoyanov*, G. P. Mylonas, M. Lerotic and G.-Z. Yang, "Intra-operative Visualizations: Perceptual Fidelity and Human Factors", IEEE/OSA Int J Disp Tech, 2008.

18. Daniel J. Riskin, Michael T., Longaker, Michael Gertner, and Thomas M. Krummel, Innovation in Surgery A Historical Perspective. Ann Surg. 2006, November; 244(5): 686–693.

19. David TE. Innovation in surgery. *J Thorac Cardiovasc Surg.* 2000;119(suppl):38–41.

20. Denis JL, Hebert Y, Langley A, et al. Explaining diffusion patterns for complex health care innovations. *Health Care Manage Rev.* 2002;27:60–73.

21. Directive 2001/20/EC of the European Parliament and of the Council of 4 April 2001 on the approximation of the laws, regulations and administrative provisions of the Member States relating to the implementation of good clinical practice in the conduct of clinical trials on medicinal products for human use. *Official J Eur Commun* 121: 33-44.

22. Drucker P. *Innovation and Entrepreneurship.* New York: Harper & Row, 1985.

23. Dubois F, Berthelot G, Levard H. Laparoscopic cholecystectomy: historic perspective and personal experience. *Surg Laparosc Endosc.* 1991;1:52–57.

24.Dubois FP, Berthelot G. Coelioscopic cholecystectomy: preliminary report of 36 cases. *Ann Surg.* 1990;211:60–62.

25. Erik Jippes, Marjolein C. Achterkamp, Paul L.P. Brand, Derk-Jan Kiewiet, Jan Pols and Jo M.L. van Engelen. Disseminating Educational Innovations In Health-Care Practice: Training Versus Social Networks Social Science & Medicine, Volume 65, Issue 9, November 2007, Pages 1915-1927

26. European Research Council (2005) "ESF Forward Look on Nanomedicine" *An ESF - European Medical Research Councils. (EMRC) Forward Look report*

27. Filipi CJ, Fitzgibbons RJ, Salerno GM. Historical review: diagnostic laparoscopy to laparoscopic cholecystectomy and beyond. *Surg Laparosc*. 1991;3:21.

28. Freudenthal A, Samset E, Gersak B, Declerck J, Schmalsieg D, Casciaro S, Rident O, Vander Sloten J; "Augmented Reality in Surgery ARIS*ER, Research Training Network for Minimally Invasive Therapy Technologies", Endoscopic Review, Vol. 10, May 2005, No. 23:(5-10)

29. *G. Megali*, V. Ferrari, C. Freschi, B. Morabito, F. Cavallo, G. Turini, E. Troia, C. Cappelli, A. Pietrabissa, O. Tonet, A. Cuschieri, P. Dario, F. Mosca: "EndoCAS navigator platform: a common platform for computer and robotic assistance in minimally invasive surgery", Int J Med Rob Comp Ass Surg, September 2008, Vol. 4, Issue 3: 242-251,.

30. Gorden A. *The History and Development of Endoscopic Surgery.* London: Saunders, 1993.

31. Gotz F, et al. The history of laparoscopy. In: *Color Atlas of Laparoscopic Surgery.* New York: 1993.

32. Greenhalgh, T., Stones, R. Theorising big IT programmes in healthcare: Strong structuration theory meets actor-network theory, Social Science & Medicine (2010), doi: 10.1016/ j.socscimed.2009.12.034

33. Greer AL. Scientific knowledge and social consensus. *Controlled Clin Trials.* 1994;15:431–436.

34. Hanseth, O. and E. Monteiro (1997): Inscribing Behavior in Information Infrastructure Standards. <i>Accounting, Management and Information Technologies</i>, vol. 7, no. 4, pp. 183-211.

35. Helen Cooper, Robert Geyer. Using 'complexity' for improving educational research in health care. Social Science & Medicine, Volume 67, Issue 1, July 2008, Pages 177-182

36. *History of Technology*. Encyclopaedia Britannica. 2004.

37. Jippes, E., Achterkamp, M.C., Brand, P.L.P., Kiewiet, D.-J., Pols, J., van Engelen, J.M.L. Disseminating Educational Innovations In Health-Care Practice: Training Versus Social Networks, Social Science & Medicine (2010), doi: 10.1016/j.socscimed.2009.12.035

38. Jones JW, McCullough LB, Richman BW. Ethics of surgical innovation to treat rare diseases. *J Vasc Surg*. 2004;39:918–919

39. Kalbasi H, Moddaressi Y. History and development of laparoscopic surgery. *J Assoc Iranian Endosc Surgeons*. 2001;1:1.

40. Lau WY, Leow CK, Li AK. History of endoscopic and laparoscopic surgery. *World J Surg*. 1997;21:444–453.

41.Litynski GS. Endoscopic surgery: the history, the pioneers. *World J Surg*. 1999;23:745–753.

42. Lumley T. Network meta-analysis for indirect treatment comparisons. Statistics in Medicine. 2002;21:2313–2324.

43. Mancuso S. Endoscopy in gynecology. *Rays*. 1998;23:603–604.

44.*Marco Maria Lirici, Alberto Arezzo*. Surgery without scars: The new frontier of minimally invasive surgery? Controversies, concerns and expectations in advanced operative endoscopy. Minimally Invasive Therapy & Allied Technologies, 2006, Vol. 15, No. 6 : Pages 323-324

45. Marescaux J, Leroy J, Gagner M, Rubino F, Mutter D, Vix M, Butner SE, Smith MK. Transatlantic robot-assisted telesurgery. Nature 2001;413:379-80.

46. Martin Allgöwer. History and Future of the International Society of Surgery, World J. Surg. 2003, 27: 373

47. Melzer A; Technology in the operating room of the future--integration of imaging into image guided surgery,. Zentralbl Chir. 2008 Jun;133(3):197-200

48. Modlin IM, Kidd M, Lye KD. From the lumen to the laparoscope. *Arch Surg.* 2004;139:1110–1126.

49 Nasseri, B.A., Ogawa, K., Vacanti, J.P. (2001) "Tissue-Engineering: An Evolving 21st-Century Science to provide Biologic Replacement for Reconstruction and Transplantation" *Surgery 130, 781-784*

50. *Nathan Clumeck, Christine Katlama*   Call for network of Centres of Excellence in clinical research in Europe , THE LANCET March 13, 2004, Vol 363: 901 – 902.

51. Nezhat C. Videolaseroscopy and laser laparoscopy in gynaecology. *Br J Hosp Med.* 1987;38:219–224.

52. *P. Valdastri, C. Quaglia, E. Susilo, A. Menciassi, C. N. Ho, G. Anhöck, M.O. Schurr.* Wireless therapeutic endoscopic capsule: in vivo experiment, Endoscopy 2008; 40:1-4

53. Paolucci B, Schaeff B, Stuttgart G. *Gasless Laparoscopy in General Surgery and Gynecology: Diagnostic and Operative Procedures.* 1996.

54. Picard JF. American patronage and French Medicine: from the Rockefeller philanthropy to INSERM. In: *John Shaw Billings Society for the History of Medicine.* 1995.

55. R. Pugliese, M. Bailey. Laparoscopic surgery: the need of training centres to spread knowledge Journal of Medicine and The Person, December 2008, vol.6, 4: 160-163

56.REPORT OF THE NCE STEERING COMMITTEE 2008 – 2009. Government of Canada, Natural Sciences and Engineering Research Council of Canada   Canadian Institutes of Health Research Social Sciences and Humanities Research Council of Canada

57. Reynolds W Jr. The first laparoscopic cholecystectomy. JSLS. 2001 Jan- Mar, 5(1): 89 – 94.

58. Roberts EB. *Innovation: Driving Product, Process, and Market Change.* San Francisco: Jossey-Bass, 2002.

59. Rosin D. History. In: *Minimal Access Medicine and Surgery*. Oxford: Radcliffe Medical, 1993:1–9.

60. SAGES. Framework for post-residency surgical education & training. Surg Endosc 1994.8(9): 1137-1142,

61. Satava RM. Surgical robotics: the early chronicles: a personal historical perspective. Surg Laparosc Endosc Percut Tech 2002;12:6-16.

62. Schon DA. *The Reflective Practitioner: How Professionals Think in Action.* New York: Basic Books, 1983.

63. Sergio Casciaro; Minimally Invasive Technologies and Nanosystems for Diagnosis and Therapies, *Eigil Samset, 2008*

64. Shah J. Endoscopy through the ages. *Br J Urol Int.* 2002;89:645.

65. Shannon L Sibbald, Peter A. Singer, Ross Upshur, Douglas K Martin. Priority setting: what constitutes success? A conceptual framework for successful priority setting *BMC Health Services Research* 2009, 9:43

66. Shio Miyamoto, Madoka Sugiura, Shigeru Watanabe, Kunio Oyama. Development of Minimally Invasive Surgery Systems, Hitachi Review Vol. 52 (2003), No. 4:189

67. Sircus W. Milestones in the evolution of endoscopy: a short history. *J R Coll Physicians (Edinb).* 2003;33:124–13.

68. Smith PG, Reinertsen DG. *Developing Products in Half the Time.* New York: Van Nostrand Reinhold, 1991.

69. Spaner SJ, Warnock GL. A brief history of endoscopy, laparoscopy, and laparoscopic surgery. *J Laparoendosc Adv Surg Tech.* 1997;7:369–373.

70. Stirrat G, Ramsay B. Surgical innovation under scrutiny. *Lancet.* 1993;342:187–188.

71. Stirratt G, et al. The challenge of evaluating surgical procedures. *Ann R Coll Surg Engl.* 1992;74:80–84.

72. *The American Heritage Dictionary of the English Language*, 4th ed. Houghton Mifflin, 2004.

73. Tiny medical implant developed in Tuebingen, Microtechnologies from the European VECTOR project facilitate early detection of acute bleeding in the digestive tract, 2008, Novineon GmbH

74. Treuting R. Minimally invasive orthopedic surgery: arthroscopy. *Ochsner J.* 2000;2:158–163.

75. Trisha Greenhalgh, Rob Stones. Theorising big IT programmes in healthcare: Strong structuration theory meets actor-network theory Social Science & Medicine, Article in Press, December 2009

76. Utterback JM. *Mastering the Dynamics of Innovation*. Boston: Harvard Business School Press, 1994.

77. Von Hippel E. Lead users: a source of novel product concepts. *Manage Sci.* 1986;32:791–805.

78. Wiley W. Souba,Douglas Wayne Wilmore; Surgical Research, Academic Press, 2001

79. Yager P., Edwards, T. et al. (2006) "Microfluidic diagnostic technologies for global public health". *Nature 442 (7101), 412-418*

80. Young C, Horton R. Putting clinical trials into context. THE LANCET. 2005;366:107–108.

81. Zahava R.S. Rosenberg-Yunger, Abdallah S. Daar, Peter A. Singer, Douglas K. Martin. Healthcare sustainability and the challenges of innovation to biopharmaceuticals in Canada Health Policy. (2008), 87: 359–368.

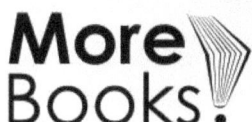
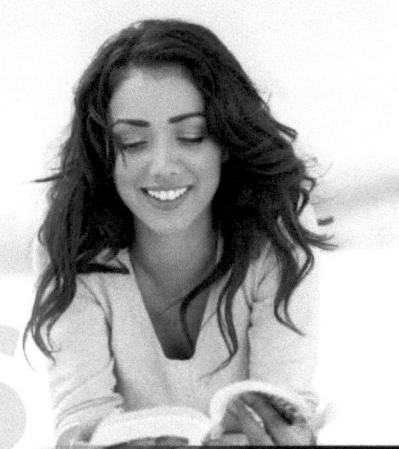

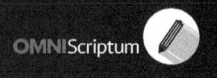

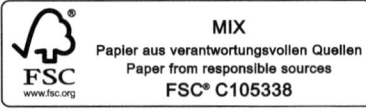
Printed by Books on Demand GmbH, Norderstedt / Germany